Movement Experiment

30 Days to Finding How You Love to Move!

Jessica Wallaker

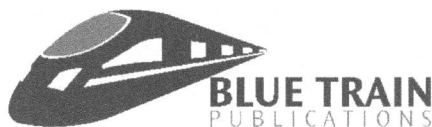

BLUE TRAIN
PUBLICATIONS

Published by Blue Train Publications in 2017

First Edition; First Printing

© 2017 Jessica Wallaker

Rcksldgym.com

Cover background image from Thobar BIGS Design

ISBN **978-0-9996436-1-7**

Dedication

I dedicate this book to you! As you go through this, my hope is that you enjoy the experience and aren't too hard on yourself. Finding YOUR movement and what works best for you is an amazing and freeing experience. I hope you have as much fun with it as I did.

Here we go!

What to do

- This is supposed to be fun! So make sure you come into this with an open mind and pure curiosity. No regrets, negative thinking; this is just an experiment. So here's how it works!

- Use each day and finish through for 30 days. Even if you skip a day or 2, just practice keeping track of how you're feeling and any other areas you can fill out.

- Start with putting down how much sleep you get, then circle either "Rested" or "Tired". This will help you find out what's working during the day and then also how much sleep YOU need.

- Since this is an experiment, see what happens when you take some time for you in the morning. It could be your main movement for the day, coffee and reading, a nice walk outside, etc. See what happens if you work to add that in as well.

- "Today's Movement" is meant for your main, designated movement. This is when you are consciously making an effort for your movement. This can be an aerobics class, swimming, CrossFit, weight lifting, biking, rock climbing, hiking, video, etc. Whatever movement you want to track that you will truly enjoy. Write down the "workout" and answer the questions at the bottom. This will help if you are experimenting and trying different things out, helping you remember what all you liked.

- The other page is for "Extra Movement". This is for your non-designated movement. Examples of this would be laps around the office, taking the stairs instead of the escalator, parking at the end of the parking lot, walking instead of driving, etc. Again, just another way to keep track of all the extra little add ins that you are doing.

- The last bit of the page is just answering the questions at the end of the day. "What did you notice today?", "Were you more productive/ have enough energy?", "Were there any stressors or excuses today?"

- At the end of the week, go back and review. Write down your thoughts of the week, good and bad so you know moving forward what's going on. Be honest, this is for you!

- This journal is to help you find out what works best for your life, schedule, situation, or time you're in. Life isn't always going to be ideal or perfect. So by filling out this journal for the next 30 days, you will have a much more clear picture of what is going to be ideal and enjoyable for you here and now.

- So go out, explore, have fun and try to see movement in more ways than just one!

Move it!

If you always put limit on everything you do, physical or anything else, it will spread into your work and into your life. There are no limits. There are only plateaus, and you must not stay there, you must go beyond them.

Bruce Lee

What I would love to see happen in the next 30 days and why

_____

_____

_____

_____

_____

_____

_____

_____

_____

_____

_____

_____

_____

_____

_____

_____

_____

_____

_____

___/ ___/ ____

Sleep:___ **Rested** or **Tired**

Did you take some time for you this am? **Y** or **N**

What did you do? Would you do it again? **Y** or **N**

_____

_____

_____

_____

Today's Movement

What did you like about this?

Would you do it again? **Y** or **N**

Extra Movement

What did you notice today?

_____

_____

_____

_____

Were you more productive/ had enough energy?

_____

_____

_____

_____

Were there any stressors or excuses today?

_____

_____

_____

___/ ___/ ___

Sleep:___ **Rested** or **Tired**

Did you take some time for you this am? **Y** or **N**

What did you do? Would you do it again? **Y** or **N**

_____

_____

_____

_____

Today's Movement

What did you like about this?

Would you do it again? **Y** or **N**

Extra Movement

What did you notice today?

_____

_____

_____

_____

Were you more productive/ had enough energy?

_____

_____

_____

_____

Were there any stressors or excuses today?

_____

_____

_____

___/ ___/ ___

Sleep:___ **Rested** or **Tired**

Did you take some time for you this am? **Y** or **N**

What did you do? Would you do it again? **Y** or **N**

_____
_____
_____
_____

Today's Movement

What did you like about this?

Would you do it again? **Y** or **N**

Extra Movement

What did you notice today?

_____

_____

_____

_____

Were you more productive/ had enough energy?

_____

_____

_____

_____

Were there any stressors or excuses today?

_____

_____

_____

___/___/___

Sleep:___ **Rested** or **Tired**

Did you take some time for you this am? **Y** or **N**

What did you do? Would you do it again? **Y** or **N**

_____

_____

_____

_____

Today's Movement

What did you like about this?

Would you do it again? **Y** or **N**

Extra Movement

What did you notice today?

_____

_____

_____

_____

Were you more productive/ had enough energy?

_____

_____

_____

_____

Were there any stressors or excuses today?

_____

_____

_____

___/___/____

Sleep:___ **Rested** or **Tired**

Did you take some time for you this am? **Y** or **N**

What did you do? Would you do it again? **Y** or **N**

_____

_____

_____

Today's Movement

What did you like about this?

Would you do it again? **Y** or **N**

Extra Movement

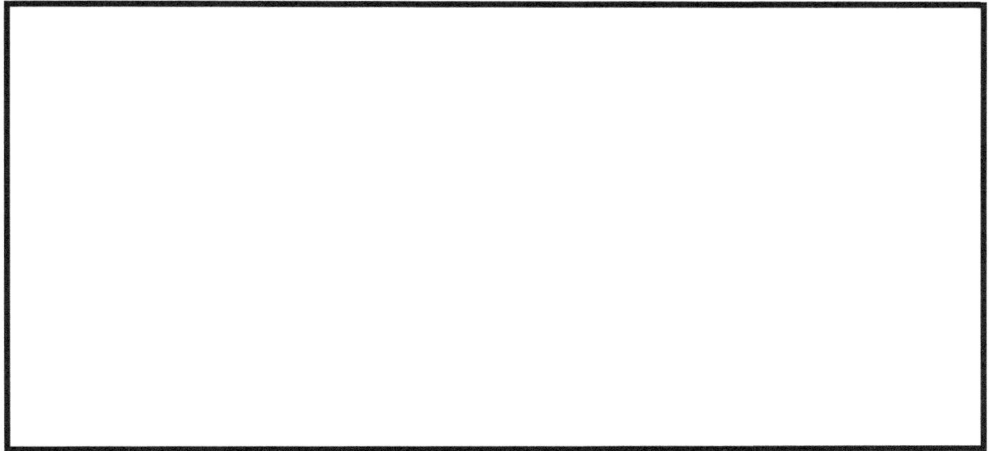

What did you notice today?

_____

_____

_____

_____

Were you more productive/ had enough energy?

_____

_____

_____

_____

Were there any stressors or excuses today?

_____

_____

_____

___/___/___

Sleep:___ **Rested** or **Tired**

Did you take some time for you this am? **Y** or **N**

What did you do? Would you do it again? **Y** or **N**

_____

_____

_____

_____

Today's Movement

What did you like about this?

Would you do it again? **Y** or **N**

Extra Movement

What did you notice today?

_____

_____

_____

_____

Were you more productive/ had enough energy?

_____

_____

_____

_____

Were there any stressors or excuses today?

_____

_____

_____

___/___/____

Sleep:___ **Rested** or **Tired**

Did you take some time for you this am? **Y** or **N**

What did you do? Would you do it again? **Y** or **N**

_____
_____
_____
_____

Today's Movement

What did you like about this?

Would you do it again? **Y** or **N**

Extra Movement

What did you notice today?

_____

_____

_____

_____

Were you more productive/ had enough energy?

_____

_____

_____

_____

Were there any stressors or excuses today?

_____

_____

_____

Week Overview

What did you find out this week?

_____

_____

_____

_____

_____

Were you surprised by anything that came up? Difficulties, limits, successes, abilities, enjoyments, etc?

_____

_____

_____

_____

_____

Any movements you enjoyed and want to try again? **Y** or **N**

If yes, what were they??

Further Thoughts

Upcoming Days Events

Any stressors you need to prep for these coming days that may affect your movement goals?

- _____
  _____

- _____
  _____

- _____
  _____

- _____
  _____

- _____
  _____

- _____
  _____

- _____
  _____

The best preparation for tomorrow is doing your best today.

H. Jackson Brown, Jr.

Final thoughts heading into the next round:

_____
_____
_____
_____
_____
_____
_____
_____
_____
_____
_____
_____
_____
_____

___/ ___/ ___

Sleep:___ **Rested** or **Tired**

Did you take some time for you this am? **Y** or **N**

What did you do? Would you do it again? **Y** or **N**

_____

_____

_____

_____

Today's Movement

What did you like about this?

Would you do it again? **Y** or **N**

Extra Movement

What did you notice today?

_____

_____

_____

_____

Were you more productive/ had enough energy?

_____

_____

_____

_____

Were there any stressors or excuses today?

_____

_____

_____

___/___/___

Sleep:___ **Rested** or **Tired**

Did you take some time for you this am? **Y** or **N**

What did you do? Would you do it again? **Y** or **N**

_____

_____

_____

_____

Today's Movement

What did you like about this?

Would you do it again? **Y** or **N**

Extra Movement

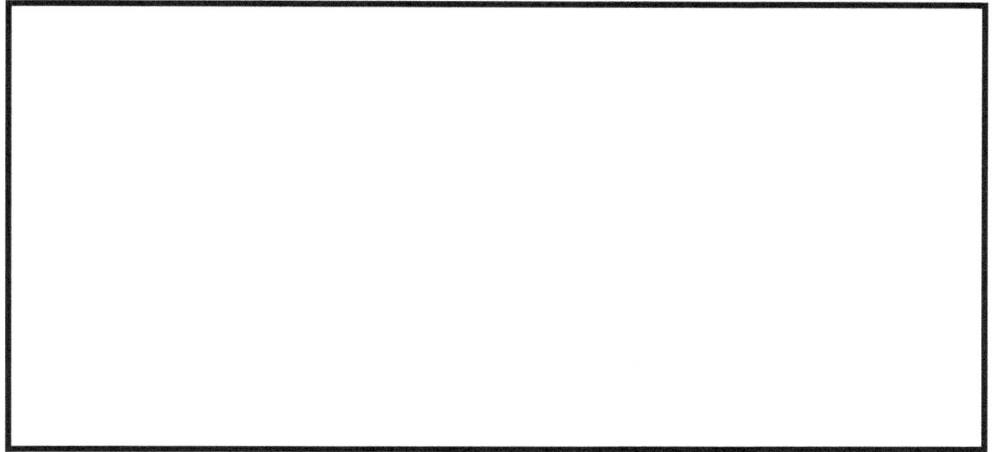

What did you notice today?

_____

_____

_____

_____

Were you more productive/ had enough energy?

_____

_____

_____

_____

Were there any stressors or excuses today?

_____

_____

_____

___/___/____

Sleep:___ **Rested** or **Tired**

Did you take some time for you this am? **Y** or **N**

What did you do? Would you do it again? **Y** or **N**

_____

_____

_____

_____

Today's Movement

What did you like about this?

Would you do it again? **Y** or **N**

Extra Movement

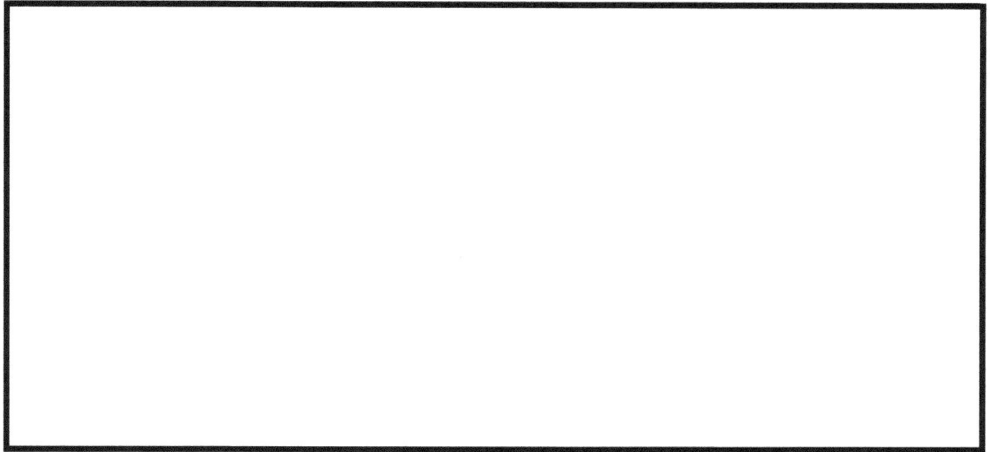

What did you notice today?

_____

_____

_____

_____

Were you more productive/ had enough energy?

_____

_____

_____

_____

Were there any stressors or excuses today?

_____

_____

_____

___/___/___

Sleep:___ **Rested** or **Tired**

Did you take some time for you this am? **Y** or **N**

What did you do? Would you do it again? **Y** or **N**

_____
_____
_____
_____

Today's Movement

What did you like about this?

Would you do it again? **Y** or **N**

Extra Movement

What did you notice today?

_____

_____

_____

_____

Were you more productive/ had enough energy?

_____

_____

_____

_____

Were there any stressors or excuses today?

_____

_____

_____

___/___/___

Sleep:___ **Rested** or **Tired**

Did you take some time for you this am? **Y** or **N**

What did you do? Would you do it again? **Y** or **N**
_____
_____
_____
_____

Today's Movement

What did you like about this?

Would you do it again? **Y** or **N**

Extra Movement

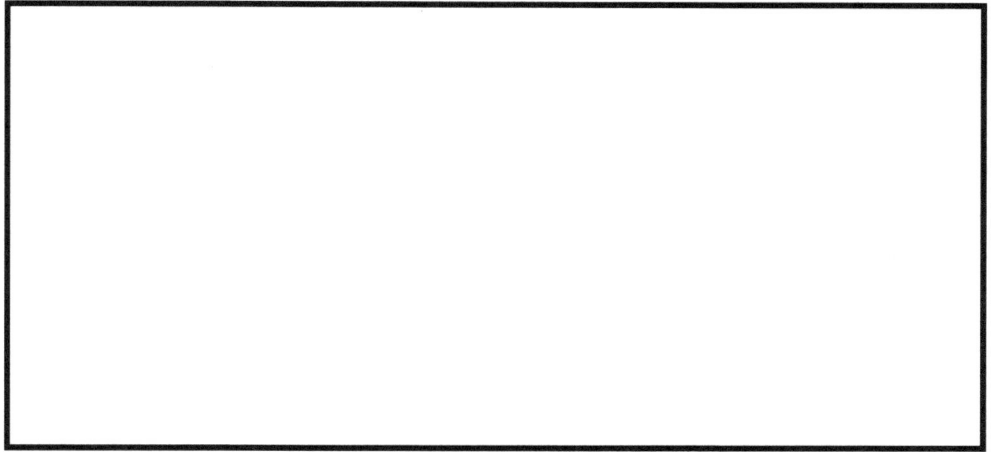

What did you notice today?

_____

_____

_____

_____

Were you more productive/ had enough energy?

_____

_____

_____

_____

Were there any stressors or excuses today?

_____

_____

_____

___/___/____

Sleep:___ **Rested** or **Tired**

Did you take some time for you this am? **Y** or **N**

What did you do? Would you do it again? **Y** or **N**

_____

_____

_____

_____

Today's Movement

What did you like about this?

Would you do it again? **Y** or **N**

Extra Movement

What did you notice today?

_____

_____

_____

_____

Were you more productive/ had enough energy?

_____

_____

_____

_____

Were there any stressors or excuses today?

_____

_____

_____

____/____/____

Sleep:____ **Rested** or **Tired**

Did you take some time for you this am? **Y** or **N**

What did you do? Would you do it again? **Y** or **N**

_____

_____

_____

_____

Today's Movement

What did you like about this?

Would you do it again? **Y** or **N**

Extra Movement

What did you notice today?

_____

_____

_____

_____

Were you more productive/ had enough energy?

_____

_____

_____

_____

Were there any stressors or excuses today?

_____

_____

_____

Week Overview

What did you find out this week?

_____

_____

_____

_____

_____

Were you surprised by anything that came up? Difficulties, limits, successes, abilities, enjoyments, etc?

_____

_____

_____

_____

_____

Any movements you enjoyed and want to try again?
Y or **N**

If yes, what were they??

Further Thoughts

Upcoming Days Events

Any stressors you need to prep for these coming days that may affect your movement goals?

- _____
  _____

- _____
  _____

- _____
  _____

- _____
  _____

- _____
  _____

- _____
  _____

- _____
  _____

Start by doing what's necessary; then do what's possible; and suddenly you are doing the impossible.

Francis of Assisi

Final thoughts heading into the next round:

_____

_____

_____

_____

_____

_____

_____

_____

_____

_____

_____

_____

___/___/___

Sleep:___ **Rested** or **Tired**

Did you take some time for you this am? **Y** or **N**

What did you do? Would you do it again? **Y** or **N**

_____

_____

_____

_____

Today's Movement

What did you like about this?

Would you do it again? **Y** or **N**

Extra Movement

What did you notice today?

_____

_____

_____

_____

Were you more productive/ had enough energy?

_____

_____

_____

_____

Were there any stressors or excuses today?

_____

_____

_____

___/___/___

Sleep:___ **Rested** or **Tired**

Did you take some time for you this am? **Y** or **N**

What did you do? Would you do it again? **Y** or **N**

_____

_____

_____

_____

Today's Movement

What did you like about this?

Would you do it again? **Y** or **N**

Extra Movement

What did you notice today?

_____

_____

_____

_____

Were you more productive/ had enough energy?

_____

_____

_____

_____

Were there any stressors or excuses today?

_____

_____

_____

___/ ___/ ___

Sleep:___ **Rested** or **Tired**

Did you take some time for you this am? **Y** or **N**

What did you do? Would you do it again? **Y** or **N**

_____
_____
_____
_____

Today's Movement

What did you like about this?
Would you do it again? **Y** or **N**

Extra Movement

What did you notice today?

_____

_____

_____

_____

Were you more productive/ had enough energy?

_____

_____

_____

_____

Were there any stressors or excuses today?

_____

_____

_____

___/ ___/ ____

Sleep:___ **Rested** or **Tired**

Did you take some time for you this am? **Y** or **N**

What did you do? Would you do it again? **Y** or **N**

_____
_____
_____
_____

Today's Movement

What did you like about this?

Would you do it again? **Y** or **N**

Extra Movement

What did you notice today?

_____

_____

_____

_____

Were you more productive/ had enough energy?

_____

_____

_____

_____

Were there any stressors or excuses today?

_____

_____

_____

___/___/___

Sleep:___ **Rested** or **Tired**

Did you take some time for you this am? **Y** or **N**

What did you do? Would you do it again? **Y** or **N**

_____

_____

_____

_____

Today's Movement

What did you like about this?
Would you do it again? Y or **N**

Extra Movement

What did you notice today?

_____

_____

_____

_____

Were you more productive/ had enough energy?

_____

_____

_____

_____

Were there any stressors or excuses today?

_____

_____

_____

___/___/___

Sleep:___ **Rested** or **Tired**

Did you take some time for you this am? **Y** or **N**

What did you do? Would you do it again? **Y** or **N**

_____

_____

_____

_____

Today's Movement

What did you like about this?

Would you do it again? **Y** or **N**

Extra Movement

What did you notice today?

_____

_____

_____

_____

Were you more productive/ had enough energy?

_____

_____

_____

_____

Were there any stressors or excuses today?

_____

_____

_____

___/___/___

Sleep:___ **Rested** or **Tired**

Did you take some time for you this am? **Y** or **N**

What did you do? Would you do it again? **Y** or **N**

_____

_____

_____

_____

Today's Movement

What did you like about this?

Would you do it again? **Y** or **N**

Extra Movement

What did you notice today?

_____

_____

_____

_____

Were you more productive/ had enough energy?

_____

_____

_____

_____

Were there any stressors or excuses today?

_____

_____

_____

Week Overview

What did you find out this week?

_____

_____

_____

_____

_____

Were you surprised by anything that came up? Difficulties, limits, successes, abilities, enjoyments, etc?

_____

_____

_____

_____

_____

Any movements you enjoyed and want to try again? **Y** or **N**

If yes, what were they??

Further Thoughts

_____

_____

_____

_____

_____

_____

_____

_____

_____

_____

_____

_____

_____

_____

_____

_____

_____

_____

Upcoming Days Events

Any stressors you need to prep for these coming days that may affect your movement goals?

- _____
  _____
- _____
  _____
- _____
  _____
- _____
  _____
- _____
  _____
- _____
  _____
- _____
  _____

Change your thoughts and you change your world.

Norman Vincent Peale

Final thoughts heading into the next round:

_____

_____

_____

_____

_____

_____

_____

_____

_____

_____

_____

_____

_____

___/ ___/ ___

Sleep:___ **Rested** or **Tired**

Did you take some time for you this am? **Y** or **N**

What did you do? Would you do it again? **Y** or **N**

_____

_____

_____

_____

Today's Movement

What did you like about this?

Would you do it again? **Y** or **N**

Extra Movement

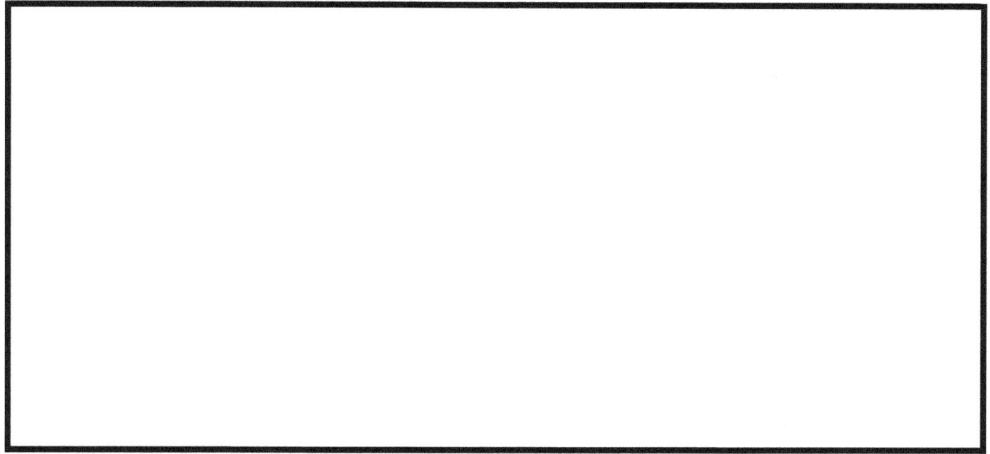

What did you notice today?

_____

_____

_____

_____

Were you more productive/ had enough energy?

_____

_____

_____

_____

Were there any stressors or excuses today?

_____

_____

_____

___/___/___

Sleep:___ **Rested** or **Tired**

Did you take some time for you this am? **Y** or **N**

What did you do? Would you do it again? **Y** or **N**

_____

_____

_____

_____

Today's Movement

What did you like about this?

Would you do it again? **Y** or **N**

Extra Movement

What did you notice today?

_____

_____

_____

_____

Were you more productive/ had enough energy?

_____

_____

_____

_____

Were there any stressors or excuses today?

_____

_____

_____

___/ ___/ ___

Sleep:___ **Rested** or **Tired**

Did you take some time for you this am? **Y** or **N**

What did you do? Would you do it again? **Y** or **N**

_____

_____

_____

_____

Today's Movement

What did you like about this?

Would you do it again? **Y** or **N**

Extra Movement

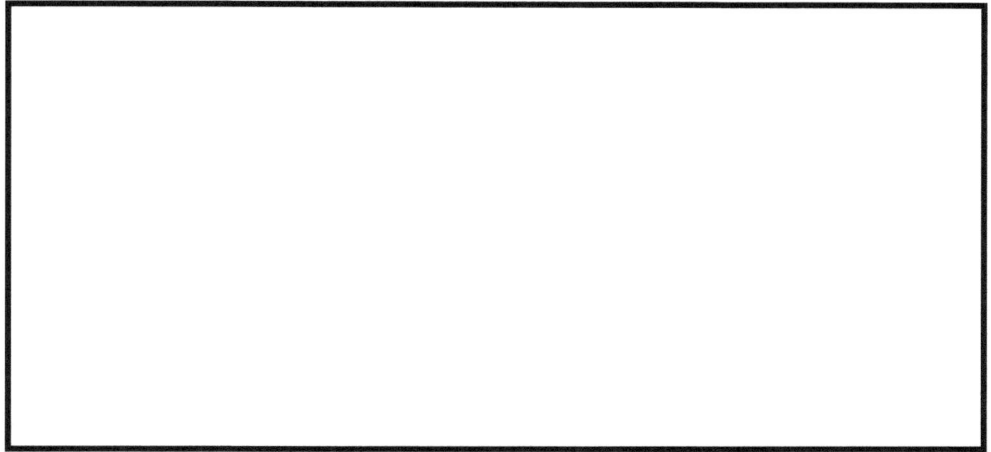

What did you notice today?

_____

_____

_____

_____

Were you more productive/ had enough energy?

_____

_____

_____

_____

Were there any stressors or excuses today?

_____

_____

_____

___/ ___/ ___

Sleep:___ **Rested** or **Tired**

Did you take some time for you this am? **Y** or **N**

What did you do? Would you do it again? **Y** or **N**

_____

_____

_____

_____

Today's Movement

What did you like about this?

Would you do it again? **Y** or **N**

Extra Movement

What did you notice today?

_____

_____

_____

_____

Were you more productive/ had enough energy?

_____

_____

_____

_____

Were there any stressors or excuses today?

_____

_____

_____

___/___/___

Sleep:___ **Rested** or **Tired**

Did you take some time for you this am? **Y** or **N**

What did you do? Would you do it again? **Y** or **N**

_____
_____
_____
_____

Today's Movement

What did you like about this?

Would you do it again? **Y** or **N**

Extra Movement

What did you notice today?

_____

_____

_____

_____

Were you more productive/ had enough energy?

_____

_____

_____

_____

Were there any stressors or excuses today?

_____

_____

_____

___/___/___

Sleep:___ **Rested** or **Tired**

Did you take some time for you this am? **Y** or **N**

What did you do? Would you do it again? **Y** or **N**

_____

_____

_____

_____

Today's Movement

What did you like about this?

Would you do it again? **Y** or **N**

Extra Movement

What did you notice today?

_____

_____

_____

_____

Were you more productive/ had enough energy?

_____

_____

_____

_____

Were there any stressors or excuses today?

_____

_____

_____

___/ ___/ ____

Sleep:___ **Rested** or **Tired**

Did you take some time for you this am? **Y** or **N**

What did you do? Would you do it again? **Y** or **N**

_____

_____

_____

_____

Today's Movement

What did you like about this?

Would you do it again? **Y** or **N**

Extra Movement

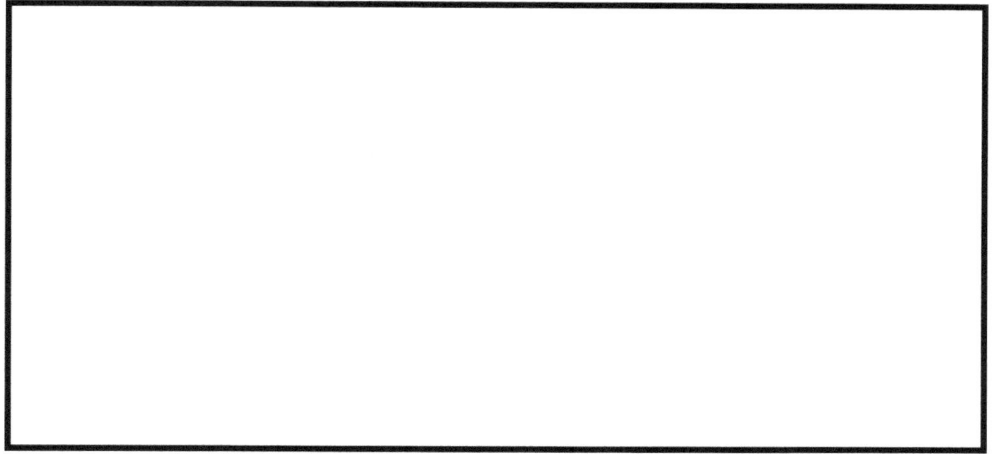

What did you notice today?

_____

_____

_____

_____

Were you more productive/ had enough energy?

_____

_____

_____

_____

Were there any stressors or excuses today?

_____

_____

_____

Week Overview

What did you find out this week?

_____

_____

_____

_____

_____

Were you surprised by anything that came up? Difficulties, limits, successes, abilities, enjoyments, etc?

_____

_____

_____

_____

_____

Any movements you enjoyed and want to try again?
Y or **N**

If yes, what were they??

Further Thoughts

_____
_____
_____
_____
_____
_____
_____
_____
_____
_____
_____
_____
_____
_____
_____
_____
_____
_____
_____
_____

Upcoming Days Events

Any stressors you need to prep for these coming days that may affect your movement goals?

- _____
  _____

- _____
  _____

- _____
  _____

- _____
  _____

- _____
  _____

- _____
  _____

- _____
  _____

What lies behind you and what lies in front of you, pales in comparison to what lies inside of you.

Ralph Waldo Emerson

Final thoughts heading into the next round:

_____

_____

_____

_____

_____

_____

_____

_____

_____

_____

_____

_____

_____

_____

____/____/____

Sleep:____ **Rested** or **Tired**

Did you take some time for you this am? **Y** or **N**

What did you do? Would you do it again? **Y** or **N**

_____

_____

_____

_____

Today's Movement

What did you like about this?

Would you do it again? **Y** or **N**

Extra Movement

What did you notice today?

_____

_____

_____

_____

Were you more productive/ had enough energy?

_____

_____

_____

_____

Were there any stressors or excuses today?

_____

_____

_____

___/ ___/ ____

Sleep:___ **Rested** or **Tired**

Did you take some time for you this am? **Y** or **N**

What did you do? Would you do it again? **Y** or **N**

_____
_____
_____
_____

Today's Movement

What did you like about this?

Would you do it again? **Y** or **N**

Extra Movement

What did you notice today?

_____

_____

_____

_____

Were you more productive/ had enough energy?

_____

_____

_____

_____

Were there any stressors or excuses today?

_____

_____

_____

30 Days!

You made it to the end of your 30 days! What have you found out about yourself?

_____

_____

_____

_____

_____

Were you surprised by the movements your body enjoys?

_____

_____

_____

_____

_____

Was this beneficial for you? **Y** or **N**

Overall Thoughts

Next Step

There will be spots to finish out the week, so do that and then come back. Bonus!

NOW:

Is this something you feel you can keep going with?

_____

_____

_____

_____

Are you happy and comfortable with how this fits in with your life?

_____

_____

_____

_____

_____

Is there anything that will make it hard for you to keep making progress?

_____

_____

_____

_____

_____

What will be beneficial for you to have in order to keep going forward with your goals?

_____

_____

_____

_____

_____

I have faith in you! If you've truly filled out this journal and made it to the end, however that looks for you, you finished something! And that's a great thing in itself! Don't let the fact that this is done stop you from progressing on. Do what you must to stay motivated. You've got this. Now, on to the next experiment!

~ Jessie

___/___/___

Sleep:___ **Rested** or **Tired**

Did you take some time for you this am? **Y** or **N**

What did you do? Would you do it again? **Y** or **N**

_____

_____

_____

_____

Today's Movement

What did you like about this?
Would you do it again? **Y** or **N**

Extra Movement

What did you notice today?

_____

_____

_____

_____

Were you more productive/ had enough energy?

_____

_____

_____

_____

Were there any stressors or excuses today?

_____

_____

_____

___/ ___/ ___

Sleep:___ **Rested** or **Tired**

Did you take some time for you this am? **Y** or **N**

What did you do? Would you do it again? **Y** or **N**

_____

_____

_____

_____

Today's Movement

What did you like about this?

Would you do it again? **Y** or **N**

Extra Movement

What did you notice today?

_____

_____

_____

_____

Were you more productive/ had enough energy?

_____

_____

_____

_____

Were there any stressors or excuses today?

_____

_____

_____

___/___/___

Sleep:___ **Rested** or **Tired**

Did you take some time for you this am? **Y** or **N**

What did you do? Would you do it again? **Y** or **N**

_____

_____

_____

_____

Today's Movement

What did you like about this?

Would you do it again? **Y** or **N**

Extra Movement

What did you notice today?

_____

_____

_____

_____

Were you more productive/ had enough energy?

_____

_____

_____

_____

Were there any stressors or excuses today?

_____

_____

_____

___/ ___/ ___

Sleep:___ **Rested** or **Tired**

Did you take some time for you this am? **Y** or **N**

What did you do? Would you do it again? **Y** or **N**

_____

_____

_____

_____

Today's Movement

What did you like about this?

Would you do it again? **Y** or **N**

Extra Movement

What did you notice today?

_____

_____

_____

_____

Were you more productive/ had enough energy?

_____

_____

_____

_____

Were there any stressors or excuses today?

_____

_____

_____

___/___/___

Sleep:___ **Rested** or **Tired**

Did you take some time for you this am? **Y** or **N**

What did you do? Would you do it again? **Y** or **N**
_____
_____
_____
_____

Today's Movement

What did you like about this?
Would you do it again? **Y** or **N**

Extra Movement

What did you notice today?

_____

_____

_____

_____

Were you more productive/ had enough energy?

_____

_____

_____

_____

Were there any stressors or excuses today?

_____

_____

_____

It is never too late to be what you might have been.

George Eliot

What I would love to see happen in the next 30 days and why

_____

_____

_____

_____

_____

_____

_____

_____

_____

_____

_____

_____

_____

_____

_____

_____

_____

_____

_____

About the Author

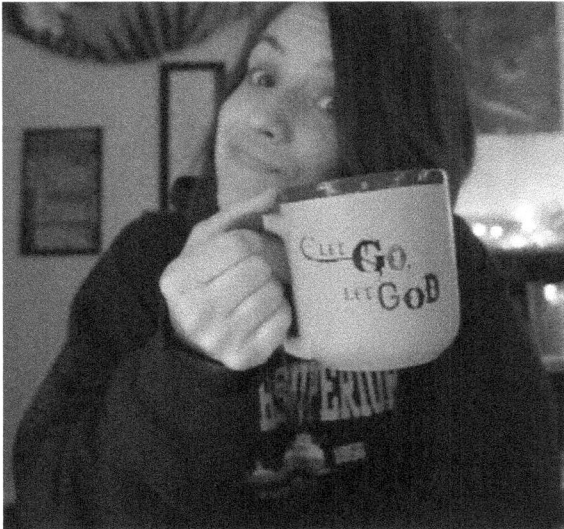

Confident and Fit Coaching
rcksldgym.com

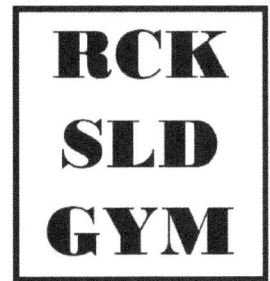

RCK
SLD
GYM

Jessica Wallaker is a young entrepreneur in the making. From starting her own coaching business, Confident and Fit Coaching, in her early 20's to writing her first journal in 2017. Her main goal with coaching and writing is to help people better understand what it is that they want to get out of their life. Showing them that health doesn't have to be one separate compartment in their hectic schedule; it can be fun, enjoyable and also stress free. Who would've thought!

If you are interested in any coaching or upcoming programs, please go to rcksldgym.com

So be sure to follow her on social media or check out her website to keep up-to-date on all the new adventures and endeavors she is trying out today.

Also By Jessica Wallaker

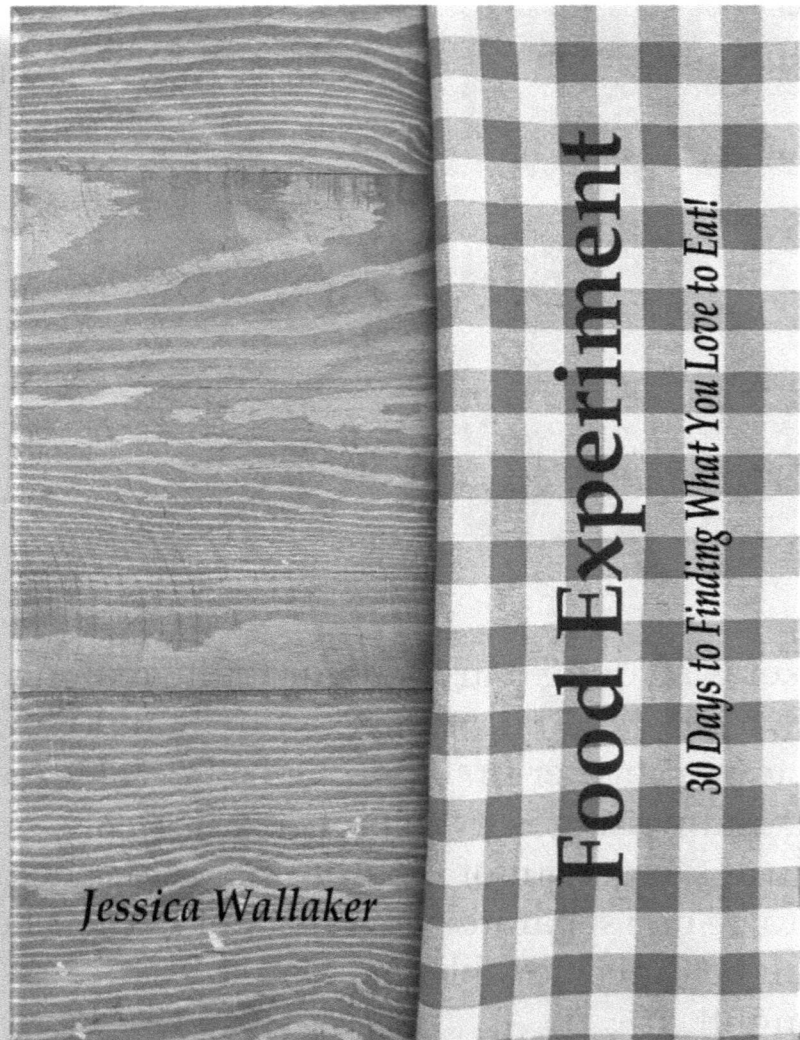

Jessica Wallaker

Food Experiment

30 Days to Finding What You Love to Eat!

Available at amazon.com
Be sure to check us out at rcksldgym.com for new additions
coming soon!

www.ingramcontent.com/pod-product-compliance
Lightning Source LLC
Chambersburg PA
CBHW080208300326
41934CB00038B/3408